Carb Cycling Diet

Table of Contents

Introduction

I want to thank you and congratulate you for downloading the book, *"Carb Cycling Diet"*

Carb cycling is truly a very interesting diet. When done the right way, you would not only enjoy the diet, but you would also achieve fast and sustainable results.

However, the key to unlock the potential benefits of carb cycling is doing it the right way. Ensure that you apply the principles you have learnt in this book and use it to develop a plan that would work for you. The recipes in this book are easy to understand and prepare, so you don't have to worry if you are not a cooking-pro because the recipes have been given to you in a step-by-step manner. When you cook your own food, it is easier to track what you are eating and you don't need to worry if you are eating right and healthy. Each of the recipes are based on the basic foundation which includes the low-carb and high-carb variations. The recipes are still customizable. You have a lot of endless possibilities in creating delicious and healthy meals.

Losing weight is not just about eating healthy foods but also eating the right portions. While there are a lot of applications that you can download to help you keep track of the amount of calories that you eat, it is still important that you know how portioning works.

Thanks again for downloading this book, I hope you enjoy it!

Chapter 1 History of carb cycling

Those who have been trying to lose excess pounds are probably familiar with the more popular diet fads, diet craze and diet menu plans. These diet plans' popularity stems from their promise of helping users to lose weight fast. These plans have different concepts and attacks.

Among the most recognizable are the low-carb diet plans that promise people that they will receive immediate positive results. However, some of those who tried these types of diet plans reported gaining the weight they lost right after reintroducing carbohydrates into their diets.

From popular trainer and transformation specialist, Chris Powell, comes carb cycling, a diet plan that alternates high-carb and low-carb days. How is it different from all the other weight loss plans before it?

There was a time in the 1970s and 1980s called the 'highcarb mania'. Most of the popular diets of that time encouraged the intake of large amounts of carbohydrates. However, this perception changed drastically in the 1990s and an exact opposite became popular. The diets of the 1990s, and later, concentrated on reducing the carbohydrate in the diet, giving rise to the 'lowcarb mania'. With that said, people are still unclear about how the carbs are used up in the human body. More precisely, the contribution of carb amounts to any weight loss program needs to be understood. Without any understatement, it can be said that your carb intake can be the game changer in your weight loss program and be responsible for weight loss.

On the other hand, it might just be the macronutrient that can destroy your plan completely. Today, the scenario has changed and there are a plethora of resources available for people to study and know what their bodies are going through, with and without a weight loss regime. Despite this availability of resources, people are still facing weight issues so much so that obesity is one of the most common problems faced by the world today.

This brings us to question as to why the scenario is deteriorating. After much contemplation, experts have stated that the reason behind the increasing problem of obesity is that none of the existing fitness systems understands the functioning of the human body. Most of the existing dietary approaches end up lowering the body's metabolism. As a result, the body loses all its energy and motivation to lose weight.

Franco Carlotto created carb cycle regiment in the 1990s, in his attempt to prepare for the Mr. World Fitness Title. In the process, he also helped millions of people around the world in maintaining a lean and healthy body. The main objective of this dietary approach was to help people achieve not just their long-term weight loss goals, but to reach both the short-term and long-term milestones in time. This technique has been developed from the analysis of how our ancestors ate and depleted their carb storage to maintain a healthy body. Although, the times have changed, the human body and the way it functions remains the same.

Therefore, the solution to weight loss issues also remains the same in the 21st century. We have to understand and manipulate our own carb storage system to get the weight loss results we expect. The carb cycle approach requires an individual to alternate high carb and low carb cycles on a daily basis, regulating the natural storage system of the body in such a way that the body doesn't store anything and burns more than what is expected on a daily and weekly basis. The low carb days deplete the body of its carbohydrates. However, the high carb days replenish the carb reserves. In this way, the body doesn't get exhausted of its energy and resources at any time. On a personal level, you don't have to give up on all your carbohydrate rich foods altogether. You can just vary them on the

Chapter 2 what is carb cycling?

This has probably got you curious and wondering what carb cycling is all about. Carb cycling is simply an eating plan that lets you alternate between high carbs and low carbs on different days.

Your body makes use of different classes of food to perform its various functions. Protein for instance, is used for bodybuilding while carbohydrate supplies your body with the energy it needs to function. However, excess carbohydrate in the body is stored as fat therefore eating too much of carbohydrate without burning it through exercise or physical activity may increase the amount of fat in the body.

This is why some people choose to avoid carbohydrates altogether. However, completely avoiding carbohydrates would not do your body any good neither will it make you lose weight effectively. Although you may shed the pounds faster, there are a few downsides to that.

For one, you would be robbing your body of the essential nutrients and fiber that it needs. Also, low or no-carb diets are hardly sustainable. Therefore, it is almost impossible to achieve long-term weight loss on such diets.

Another downside of low-carb diets is that carbohydrates are actually replaced with other classes of foods like fats and proteins and this may lead to an increase in cholesterol levels thereby increasing risk of cardiovascular diseases.

There are so many other negative effects of low carb diets such as dizziness, fatigue, nausea, bad breath, and headache, which occur because of the body going into a state of ketosis.

Your body goes into a state of ketosis when you eat less than 20 grams of carbohydrates daily. Eating less than 20 grams of carbohydrates daily causes the body to switch from using carbohydrates as a source of energy to using stored fat in the body. This causes ketones to accumulate in the body and lead to the negative effects mentioned above.

On a carb cycling diet however, you do not have to cut down on carbs altogether; rather, you would control the way you consume your carbs. You would alternate your carbohydrate consumption in such a way that on some days, you eat foods that are very rich in carbohydrates while on some days, you go for foods with low carbohydrate content.

Eating this way helps to improve your metabolism so that your body begins to burn more calories. The healthy carbs, which you consume on this diet, would also help to control your blood sugar, reduce cravings, and improve your energy levels.

You do not feel weak or hungry as with other diets that have their principles based on starvation.

Carb Cycling Plans

There are four different carb cycling plans, which you should know about. They include:

Easy Carb Cycle

As a beginner, you should start with the Easy Carb Cycle. The Easy Carb Cycle is a very effective plan for people who find it hard to cut out on certain foods.

Are you the type who loves pizza so much that the thought of not having it in a week makes you dread any form of diet at all? Then the Easy Carb Cycle is for you.

This carb-cycling plan allows you to alternate between high carb and low carb days and on your high carb days; you are allowed to enjoy your favorite foods or snacks that you crave as long as you don't have them at dinner.

So yes, you can have cakes, chips, ice cream, or anything you want and still lose weight. The only rule is that you can only have these things as a REWARD MEAL on your HIGH-CARB DAYS.

Sounds easy, right? It's actually easy.

Another rule is that you have to spread your meals throughout the day. Instead of eating three heavy meals a day, you should have at least five small meals throughout the day. And this applies to both high-carb and low carb days. This further helps to boost your metabolism and helps you burn more calories.

So on an easy carb cycle, this is what your eating plan would look like:

Sunday	Reward meal	High carb day
Monday		Low carb day
Tuesday	Reward meal	High carb day
Wednesday		Low carb day

Thursday	Reward meal	High carb da
Friday		Low carb da
Saturday	Reward meal	High Carb d

Remember, if you are craving anything, anything at all, you don't have to deprive yourself; all you need to do is to move it up to your high carb day or eat it as your reward meal.

You can move up to another carb cycling plan or you can stay with this plan throughout your diet; the decision is entirely yours to make.

Classic Carb Cycle

The classic carb cycle is a step higher than the easy carb cycle but is just as easy and effective for weight loss as the easy carb cycle.

On the classic carb cycle, you are allowed one whole day to satisfy all your cravings. This day serves as your reward day. So instead of having a reward meal every other day as with the easy carb cycle, you would have one full day to satisfy all your cravings.

The good thing is that you would still be able to alternate between the high and the low carb days.

This is what your eating plan on a classic carb cycle would look like:

Sunday	Reward day
Monday	Low carb day
Tuesday	High carb day
Wednesday	Low carb day

Thursday	High carb day
Friday	Low carb day
Saturday	High carb day

On this cycle, you are able to lose weight quickly and constantly. You may also choose to remain on this cycle throughout your weight loss journey or move up to another carb-cycling plan.

Turbo Cycle

The Turbo cycle helps you lose weight faster than all the other carb cycles. Instead of alternating high carb days with low carb days as you do on other plans, on the turbo cycle, you would have to put in two low carb days for every high carb day. So, in a week you get four low carb days, two high carb days and one reward day.

This type of eating plan helps you burn fat consistently for two days before re-stoking on your high carb day.

The turbo cycle is also very powerful in the sense that you do not have to restrict your calories. Women can have at least 1,200 calories a day while men can have at least 1,500 calories daily.

This is what your eating plan on a turbo cycle would look like:

Sunday	Reward day
Monday	Low carb day
Tuesday	Low carb day
Wednesday	High carb day

Thursday	Low carb day
Friday	Low carb day
Saturday	High carb day

The turbo cycle is a powerful weight loss accelerator and you may decide to stay on this plan throughout your weight loss journey or move on to another cycle.

The Fit Cycle

The fourth carb-cycling plan is the fit cycle. This is the best carb-cycling plan for people who are highly active physically such as athletes, body builders, and trainers.

The fit cycle plan helps you eliminate fat while supplying your body with the fuel, which it needs to perform. There are only two low carb days a week in this cycle.

On the extra high carb days, your body is able to absorb more glycogen, which serves as energy for high performance. This is alternated by the low carb days when the body's supply of glycogen has been depleted and the muscles have developed insulin-sensitivity thereby allowing it to soak up more carbs and burn extra calories on the high carb and reward days.

The fit cycle eating plan would look like this:

Sunday	Reward day
Monday	High carb day
Tuesday	High carb day

Wednesday	Low carb day
Thursday	High carb day
Friday	High carb day
Saturday	Low carb day

The fit cycle allows you to lose weight and burn fat without compromising on your physical performance. You would still get all the energy you need to achieve your athletic goals while losing weight rapidly.

Chapter 3 Why carb cycle?

Carb cycling helps you structure your carb consumption in such a way that you do not eat too little so that it begins to slow down your metabolism and you do not eat too much either.

Here are a few reasons why carb cycling is the best diet for you or anyone who is really serious about losing weight the healthy way;

Carb Cycling Promotes Fat Burning

On a carb cycling diet, you would not just lose water weight as with most traditional diets; you would actually lose fat.

Carb cycling enables your body to burn fat as fuel as opposed to just burning carbohydrates and muscle tissues.

Carb Cycling Helps You Build Lean Muscles

Carb cycling also helps you to get leaner while building muscles. This is because carb cycling helps to make your body better at controlling insulin so that more glucose is stored in the muscles instead of fat cells.

Carb Cycling Increases Receptiveness to Insulin

The high carb days helps to stimulate insulin response so that nutrients are moved to your muscle cells causing them to grow while the low carb days makes your body much more responsive to insulin.

Carb Cycling Helps You Reduce Consumption of Bad Carbs

All carbs are not created equal. There are the good and healthy carbs and there are the not-so healthy ones. The unhealthy carbs increase blood glucose levels and make you hungry and crave unhealthy foods like candy, fries, and other snacks. Carb cycling helps you consume less of these unhealthy carbs and more of healthy carbs like whole grains, oats, fruits, legumes, and whole oats.

Carb Cycling is Easy

Carb cycling is not like any of the diets that leave you starving, weak, and unable to concentrate. You actually get to eat the foods you love while losing weight.

You can actually go out with your friends, go out on dinner dates, and still enjoy regular meals while you are on the diet.

What can be better than this?

How to determine if Carb Cycling is Safe for You

There's sad news here. Carb cycling works and is one of the easiest and most effective diet plans for weight loss currently.

But sadly, carb cycling is not for everyone. Carb cycling is only good for people who want to use it as a short-term approach to weight loss.

Most nutritionists and health experts advice that carb cycling should only be done for a short period of at most four months.

Doing the carb recycling diet for longer than this may affect the body negatively.

Participating in the carb cycling diet program can help you prevent sudden dips in your metabolic rate.
This diet program can help you to prevent imbalances in your digestive system. In the process, you keep yourself from feeling

bloated, regardless of the cycle of the diet program that you are currently in.

This diet program helps you to decrease the average amount of carbohydrates that you consume within a certain period of time.

Your body will not have to deal with excessive glycogen levels that will most likely not be utilized for the rest of the day. This will give your liver and your pancreas some much-needed rest. Because of this, you can prevent medical conditions such as diabetes mellitus. Some studies have also shown that decreased exposure to high glycogen levels helps to prevent cardiovascular system disorders from bring harmful.

As for leptin production, you can expect to have more as you go along with carb cycling.

Leptin is a substance that can help to regulate your hunger. Therefore, leptin can help you have decreased incidences of food cravings. In the process, you can expect your metabolism to significantly increase. This can lead to better weight management overall and the effective shedding of fat tissue.

Because of food item regulation and regular exercise, you can expect a steady boost in biochemicals, which can assist you in breaking down the fat tissue stored in your body.

While participating in this diet program, you can expect increased levels of testosterone and HGH in your body. This can help you to break down fat molecules by improving the growth rates of major muscle groups. These can also help you increase your metabolic rate for an even more effective fat breakdown process.

Helps to promote the entire process of fat loss.

Aside from fat breakdown evident through food amount and type regulation, you must make changes in your physical activity levels. Specifically, you must increase the intensity of the exercises that you perform in order to help you to develop your muscle groups. The difficulties of the workout routines that you need to perform are directly proportional to the fat breakdown potentials through carbohydrate and nutrient consumption.

In relation to the previous point, carb cycling can help you to prevent gaining more fat than allowed.

More protein means more building blocks for your major muscle groups. This can translate to larger muscle masses overall. Because your muscles will be larger, they will consume more energy sources in order to keep them going. Fat tissue is a major source of energy for these muscles. As you work out more, and consume protein, you will lose more adipose tissue. In the process, you will develop a leaner body mass.

The longer you adhere to the diet program; you can expect your glycogen restoration levels to have improvements.

Because your diet program helps with significant improvements for your major muscle groups, you can expect that these muscle groups will also use up more glycogen. This is what happens when you participate in this diet program. As your muscles get bigger, the amount of dormant energy reserves decrease. When this happens, excessive adipose tissue is eventually obliterated.

As soon as you get used to carb cycling, it will be easier for you to keep doing exercises with a high intensity.

As much as the diet program helps to increase the amount of fat that your body uses up, it is much easier for your body to pace the energy usage. In other words, there is a better distribution of energy sources when you perform physical activity. This especially holds true when you are required to perform relatively difficult exercise routines for a prolonged period of time.

Because of the promising benefit of fat breakdown, this diet program can help you to develop and maintain a lean body form.

After you have noticed the significant improvements for your body, you will notice that there are major improvements on the functionalities of your muscles overall. This can be more convenient because you can easily perform the tasks that you must do. The good news is that you get to perform these tasks even better than they were performed before.

This diet program can keep your muscles and bones from deteriorating.

As your muscles begin to develop, you will have a better chance of using them for most of your tasks. When this happens, there is a good chance of developing them by virtue of "constant pressure". Moreover, your body has a good chance of gaining the right nutrients which can help to prevent further bone and muscle deterioration.

Carb cycling can help in muscle growth and development.

Due to the fact that there is a fixed amount of minimum protein consumption that you must take for every meal, your body has a virtually unlimited supply of amino acids. Amino acids are substances that your body can use for muscle reinforcement and repair. Coupled with the right exercise, you can enjoy larger and leaner muscle mass within four to six weeks.

Unlike other diet programs out there, this program can help you to prevent adaptation over time.

Preventing adaptation over time is extremely helpful because it can help you to prevent any weight regain. Because of the unpredictability in diet and workout modifications, there comes a time in which your body will guess on what comes next.

This diet program can prevent plateaus from occurring.

Since this diet program is somewhat unpredictable, you are able to dodge the possibility of exponentially decreasing benefits and negative health impacts.

You will not experience food deprivation because of the balanced meal plans suggested.

Although it seems like food deprivation is stressed because of food choice restrictions described in the book, your body will not feel deprived because it receives a complete set of nutrients for each day. Therefore, your body will not seek more food items in the long run.

In relation to the previous point, you will have a prolonged satiety period.

Satiety takes place because most of the recommended food items included in the diet have delayed processing capacities in the stomach.

This means that these specific food items will induce a longer digestion time for your body. The stomach will send a signal to the brain that it is still full after some time. The brain will then send impulses that will tell your stomach to keep on processing the food items and absorbing the nutrients from these food items.

Food cravings will never be an issue once you take part in this diet program.

On this diet, you are exposed to decreased levels of refined carbohydrates. Refined carbs are included in those food groups in which your digestive system can easily break down. More food items will eventually lead to glycogen pile up. Fortunately, you do not have to suffer this fate if you participate in the diet program because the meal plans satisfy you and with this, you have less chance of gaining weight.

Chapter 4 how carb cycling works

Carb cycling, also known as carbohydrate cycling, is a weight management technique that requires certain meal plans to be incorporated with regulated types of food groups in them. Usually, the food items included in the meal plans are monitored for carbohydrate content. As the name of the diet program implies, carbohydrate-laden food items are important to monitor because they determine the type of food item that will be eaten for each meal on any given day.

There are different aspects to the carbohydrate cycle that you should understand.

You should keep in mind that there are six meals that you have to consume each day. Each of the meals eaten should have regular intervals between each other. This will help to ensure that you develop a regular and highly functional metabolic rate for your digestive system.

During a high carb-laden day, you are allowed to consume as many carbohydrates as you want, but only for certain meals within the day.

Out of the six meals that you will eat on that day, you may consume as many carbs as you desire for four of the meals. You may eat carbs as soon as you have consumed the recommended amount of fats and proteins.

Aside from your unlimited carbohydrate consumption, you must eat a piece of fruit with 50 to 100 calories before you consume any carbs. The fruit you consume contains fructose that will help your body to produce more energy. The body can produce more energy by virtue of glycogen storage inside your liver. Even if fructose is a form of sugar, this cannot affect the fat production in your body because the consumption of 50 to 100 calories is not enough to elicit an effect in your body. Instead, the fructose value that you consume can help promote prolonged satiety for your digestive system. Thus, you will have a decreased need to eat additional meals in between the predetermined six meals on this specific day. And, this will prevent you from overeating.

The Low- carbs day may be considered as the most complicated among the three phases of this diet program due to certain macronutrient goals that you must fulfill.

For this specific carb cycling day, you must consume carbohydrates for only three out of the six meals that you eat. Before you consume any carbohydrates, you need to include the prescribed amount of protein and fat in your diet. Moreover, you must consume a small fruit with 50 to 100 calories in it beforehand.

The recommended amount of carbohydrates is set at one gram of carbs for every one pound of weight in your body each day. After computing for the total value of carbs that you must consume each day, you would then divide this value by three. This is the amount of carbs that you are allowed to eat for three out of the six meals during your low carbs day. You should note that the amount of carbs that you need to consume for each meal should be equally distributed in order to ensure consistency in your metabolic rate.

A no-carbs day is considered the easiest, but most important, among the phases of carb cycling.

The no-carbs day is regarded as the most controversial part of the carbs cycling diet program. As the term suggests, you are not allowed to eat any food items with carbs for the six meals that you will have for that day. But, you still need to consume the minimum amount of fat and protein for all your meals to prevent delaying your muscle development process. Apart from these instructions, you may consume as much protein as you want for your meals on this day.

Initially, you may find it difficult to get through this day. One way to keep on track is to motivate yourself by thinking about the high carbs day that lies only a few days ahead.

There are numerous factors which can determine if you will emerge successful while engaging in the carbs cycling diet program.

You are able to control some of these factors of the diet program. But, you cannot manipulate the other factors of this diet because they are fixed and based on the specific genetic aspects of your body.

If you want to build a solid foundation in order to ensure success for your diet program, setting certain diet related goals can help you do this.

Your goals will determine the success rate that you will attain at the end of the diet program, once you complete the program. Experts recommend that you adhere to a set time, as well as realistic, objective, specific, and concrete goals. Composing your goals in this manner will help you to stay motivated. These goals will help you to assess your progress during the time you are on the diet.

Before you start off with the actual diet program, you should set your long term and short term goals. In the process of goal setting, you should already know what you want to attain after the program. In the long run, this will tell you how much satisfaction you will attain after reaching your goals.

Body builds are uncontrollable variables that can somehow determine your success rate in the carb cycling diet program.

Different body types have different reactions to certain diet programs that are introduced. Therefore, you must have your body type assessed in order to determine how you use the program to create significant and positive results for your body.

• Ectomorphic is known as the thin body type. People with this body type have a small and rather delicate body frame and bone structure. Experts do not usually recommend this diet program for people with ectomorphic body types because they already have high metabolic rates used to get rid of the adipose tissues in their body.

• Mesomorphic is known as the lean body type. People with this body type have naturally athletic physiques. Given this fact, mesomorphs usually manifest with large muscle groups and sturdy bone structures.

• Endomorphic is the soft and solid body type. Compared to the two previous body types presented, the endomorphic body type tends to have the largest proportions of fat. People with this body type are the most sensitive to carbohydrates. This implies that they should consume fewer carbohydrates because they tend to gain more fats compared to the mesomorphs and the ectomorphs. Given these premises, endomorphs have the most weight management benefits if they maximize the intricacies of the program.

Your lifestyle can tell you how successful you will be on this diet program even before you start.

For most diet programs out there, you must also incorporate various workout routines and physical activities into your daily schedule. This activity is important because it will set your major muscle groups to work. As soon as they are set to work, you initiate the processes of fat breakdown and muscle buildup. You must do these things for the rest of your life.

Support systems can mean a lot, especially when you are going through difficult phases of your carb cycle.

Working with a support system can make you accountable for everything that you are about to do which is related to your diet program. The right support system reminds you to fulfill your goals and plans. They can also affirm and encourage you when you are successful. If you are doing something that can benefit you in the long run, they will let you know. Some support systems can even assist you in creating diet and exercise alternatives.

Like other diet programs out there, the carb cycling diet includes different goals for each phase that you go through while in the cycle.

The main goal of this diet program is to help you lose those unwanted pounds. In the process, carb cycling should help you to develop lean muscle mass instead of wasting muscle mass. As soon as you see that you are getting rid of fats while toning up your body, you will eventually get motivated to continue the program.

Monitoring your progress as you go along the diet program can help you to further boost your motivation levels. To help you monitor your achievements while participating in the program, you have to weigh yourself and take measurements regularly, such as hip to waist ratio and waistline measurements. You must obtain baseline measurements for these aspects as these will serve as the base of comparisons for your next measurements. Afterward, you will need to take measurements every six to eight weeks that you are on the diet. On average, each cycle of this diet program lasts for three to four days.

Because workouts are considered a part of any type of effective diet program, you should make specific considerations when working out while you are involved in the carb cycling diet program.

Right after performing all your workout routines, you will have to consume 30 to 50 grams worth of protein. This will help to reinforce the process of muscle development and assist you in muscle repair. If you are on a low carbs or high carbs day, during the day of the workout, you have to follow up your protein intake with some carbohydrates. If you want to yield better results, you have to consume food items such as whey protein and oatmeal.

Chapter 6 How much to eat and of what?

What you can Include in Your Diet

Aside from the recipes above, you will have examples of carb-cycling foods that you are allowed to have:

Protein:

Beef

- Cube steak – 2.5 oz
- Low sodium roast beef - 3 oz
- Extra lean sirloin steak – 2 oz
- Lean flank steak – 2.5 oz
- Venison – 2 oz.

Dairy

- Cottage cheese ½ cup
- Egg whites – 4 whites
- Egg substitutes – 1 cup
- Plain Greek yogurt -3/4 cup

Lean Ground Meats

- Extra lean ground beef – 2 oz
- Ground chicken breast – 4 oz
- Ground turkey – 3 oz

Poultry

- Duck breast – 2 oz

- Skinless chicken thigh – 3 oz

- Skinless chicken breast – 3.5 oz

Powdered

- Whey, soy, hemp, rice – 1 scoop

Fish

- Salmon fillet – 2 oz

- Sardines – 52 g (4 sardines)

- Canned tuna – 3 oz

- Tuna fillet – 3 oz

- White fish – 2.5 oz

Shellfish

- Raw clams – 5 oz

- Shrimp/lobster – 4 oz

Vegetable Protein

- Tempeh – 2 oz

- Tofu – 4 oz

White Meat

- Pork tenderloin – 2.5 oz

Carbohydrates:
Bread

- Corn tortillas – 1 ½ servings

- Bread – 1 slice
- English muffin – ½ piece

Cereal

- Low-fat granola – ½ cup
- Old-fashioned oatmeal (cooked) – ¾ cup

Grains

- Buckwheat, Bran, Barley, Brown Rice – ½ cup
- Oats (steel-cut, cooked) – 2/3 cup
- Popcorn (no oil) – 3 cups
- Quinoa – ½ cup
- Wild rice – ½ cup

Legumes

- Beans – ½ cup
- Lentils – ½ cup
- Soybeans – ¼ cup
- Soy nuts - 3 tbsp

Pasta

- Brown rice pasta – ½ cup
- Couscous – ½ cup
- Whole grain – ½ cup

Root Vegetables

- Carrots – 2 cups

- Potatoes – ¾ cup

- Beets – 1 ½ cups

- Yams and sweet potatoes – 2/3 cup

Starchy Vegetables

- Peas – 1 cup

- Corn - 2/3 cup

Fruits:

Fresh

- Apricots – 6 pieces

- Banana – 1 piece

- Apples – 1 ½

- Berries, like blueberries, cherries, and strawberries – 1 ½ cups

- Grapes – 1 ½ cups

- Oranges – 1 piece

- Melons – 1 ½ cups

- Mangoes – 1 cup

- Lemons and limes – 5 pieces

- Papayas – 2 cups

- Plums – 3 ½ pieces

- Pineapple – ½ cup

- Peaches – 2 large pieces

- Pears – 1 piece
- Grapefruit – 1 piece
- Kiwi – 4 pieces

Vegetables:
- Asparagus – 3 ½ cups
- Artichokes – 2 pieces, medium-sized
- Broccoli – 4 cups
- Brussels sprouts – 2 ½ cups
- Bok Choy – 1 head
- Cabbage – 4 cups
- Chard – 10 leaves
- Celery – 5 cups
- Cauliflower – 4 cups
- Collard greens – 10 cups
- Eggplant – 5 cups
- Garlic – 20 cloves
- Fennel – 4 cups
- Green beans – 75 pieces
- Kale – 3 cups
- Mushrooms – 20 large pieces
- Leeks – 2 pieces
- Okra – 2 pieces medium-sized

- Radish – 5 cups

- Scallions – 10 cups

- Snow peas – 70 pods

- Parsley – 4 cups

- Spinach – 10 cups

- Tomatoes – 6 ½ pieces, medium-sized

- Turnips – 2 large pieces

- Zucchini – 2 large pieces

Fats:

Dairy:

- Cream cheese – 2 tbsp

- Egg yolk – 2

- Whip cream – 2 tbsp

- Mozzarella – 1 oz

- Parmesan – 1 oz

- Romano – 1 oz

Nuts and Seeds:

- Almonds – 1 ½ tbsp

- Peanut butter – 1 tbsp

- Pecans – 1 ½ tbsp

- Sesame seeds – 2 tbsp

- Sunflower seeds – 1 ½ tbsp

Beverages:

- Black coffee – unlimited

- Unsweetened soy milk – 1 ¼ cup

- Tea (herbal, green) – unlimited

- Water – unlimited

- Tomato juice – 2 ½ cups

Now that you have been given easy to follow and prepare carb cycling food recipes, you don't have any excuse to lose weight. Don't worry if you cannot cook all the time because of work and household chores, you can bulk-prepare your foods and store in the fridge. You can easily reheat and eat!

It is important to know some of the food items that you can incorporate in your meal plans. Some of these particular food items are included in this section.

Despite the fact that it contains fat, avocados can bring you a lot of diet related benefits.

Avocados are in fiber that which helps to flush out the harmful toxins inside your body. They also contain foliate, potassium, and monosaturated fats.

Brown rice may be a bit expensive at the store, but it can help you reap many weight loss benefits in the long run.

Brown rice is rich in dietary fiber and manganese. Manganese is considered a catalyst for carbohydrate and proteins. And, it works well with your nervous system.

Garlic is a wonder food and drug that even ancient people used.

You may incorporate garlic in your dishes if you cannot afford to eat it by itself. You may also take garlic capsules to enjoy garlic's benefits without consuming in the natural form.

Chicken serves as one of the most versatile food items that you can add into your diet.

Chicken contains nutrients such as vitamin B3, vitamin B6, selenium, and phosphorus. Chicken is also rich in protein and dietary fiber.

Milk is a complete food that can help with numerous health-related issues.

Milk can contribute to a stronger immune system, increased bone strength, and smoother skin, to name only a few benefits. Milk can also help people who are dealing with chronic illnesses.

Forbidden Foods on the Carb Cycling Diet

Although these foods are forbidden, you can have them on your cheat/reward days;

- Refined or processed carbohydrates

- Brown sugar

- Corn syrup

- Raw sugar

- Ice cream

- Chocolates

- Candy

- Soda

- Refined/white flour

- Cake

- Cookies

- Pastries

- Donuts

- Crackers

- White bread

- White rice

- Chips

- Fried meals

- Hydrogenated oils

- Alcoholic beverages like wine and beer.

- Foods high in sodium

- Artificial sweeteners like saccharin, aspartame, and sucralose.

Chapter 7 Recipes

Breakfast Recipes
Easy Breakfast Omelet

This is a great and healthy way to start your day. Eggs are among the richest sources of protein and these are inexpensive, too. Make a high-carb breakfast by mixing in fruits, whole grain toast, or oatmeal. You can prepare this for lunch or dinner and change the ratios depending on whether you are on a high-carb or low-carb day.

Ingredients:

- 4 egg whites

- 1 medium onion, chopped

- 1 medium bell pepper, chopped

- Mushrooms, chopped

- 1 medium tomato, chopped

- Spinach

- Olive oil in spray bottle

- A dash of salt and pepper or low –sodium seasoning blend

Note: You can make use of any other filling that you like. This makes 1 serving, if you want more, double the portions accordingly.

Procedure:

1. In a small bowl, whisk the egg whites for at least 45 seconds.

2. Add the vegetables and mix.

3. Spray olive oil on a non-stick pan and set to medium to high heat.

4. Add the egg whites and the veggie mixture into the pan. Season.

5. Let the omelet to finish cooking on one side and flip over to the other side with a spatula, to let it cook.

Healthy and Delicious Burrito

Ingredients:

- 6 egg whites

- 4 tbsp ground turkey

- 2 handfuls spinach

- 2-4 leaves romaine lettuce

- 2 tbsp salsa

- Vegetable oil in spray bottle

- A dash of salt and pepper

Note: This makes 2 servings, double the recipe if you want more.

Procedure:

1. Spray oil in a non-stick pan and set to medium heat.

2. Cook turkey in oil. Set aside.

3. In a large mixing bowl, beat egg whites.

4. Using another non-stick pan, spray vegetable oil and set to medium to high heat. Cook the egg in the pan. As the egg begins to set, add in the turkey and spinach. Season. Let it cook further.

5. When cooked, wrap the turkey, egg and spinach combo in two or four leaves of romaine lettuce.

6. Garnish with the salsa and roll it up.

Low-Carb Breakfast Tacos

Ingredients:

- 4 egg whites

- Corn tortillas

- 3 tomatoes, sliced

- 3 tbsp salsa

- A dash of low-sodium spice blend

- Oil in spray bottle

Note: This recipe makes 1 serving, double if you want to or adjust ingredients according to what you need.

Procedure:

1. Spray oil onto a non-stick pan. Set to medium heat.

2. Whisk the egg whites.

3. Season with the spice blend.

4. Cook until you get your preferred "scrambled" consistency.

5. Serve with corn tortillas.

6. Add in salsa and tomato slices.

Delicious Breakfast Burrito

Ingredients:

- 1 tsp canola oil

- ¼ cup onions, chopped

- 2 egg whites, whisked

- 1 low-carb high fiber tortilla

- A pinch of salt

- A pinch of pepper

- Salsa

Note: This makes 1 serving of breakfast burrito. Adjust portions accordingly.

Procedure:

- Set a non-stick pan to medium heat and cook the onions until soft.

- Season with salt and pepper.

- Add in beaten egg whites. Cook until almost set. Set aside.

- Warm tortilla in a dry pan. Pour in cooked eggs on top of the tortilla.

- Add salsa.

- Roll up and eat.

High-Carb Egg Muffin Special

Ingredients:

- 8 egg whites

- 4 slices of tomatoes

- 2 toasted English muffins

- A dash of low-sodium spice blend

Note: This recipe is good for a double-serving, add portions accordingly if you want to make more.

Procedure:

1. Whisk egg whites in a mixing bowl.

2. Spray oil in a non-stick pan. Set over medium to high heat.

3. Add the beaten eggs to the pan. Cook.

4. Add the sliced tomatoes and cooked eggs on the toasted muffin.

5. Season.

Your Favorite Breakfast Ham Omelet

Ingredients:

- 3 egg whites, whisked

- 2 tbsp low-sodium ham, chopped

- 1 tbsp onions, chopped

- 1 tbsp green bell pepper, chopped

- 1 tbsp tomato, sliced

- Fresh salsa

- A portion of cheddar cheese

- A dash of salt and pepper or low-sodium spice blend

Note: This makes 1 serving, you can double the portions if you want to make it for two persons.

Procedure:

1. Heat a non-stick pan to medium-high.

2. Add the beaten egg whites. Season.

3. Let the egg whites set on one side.

4. Place the ham, onions, bell peppers and tomatoes in the middle and continue cooking. Fold in half to enclose filling.

5. Add salsa and cheese before serving.

A Healthy BLT Sandwich

This is perfect for an anytime of the day meal as it is easy to prepare. It's ready in minutes so if you are late for work or an appointment, this will be great to perk up your day.

Ingredients:

- 2 wheat bread slices, toasted

- 2 medium tomatoes, sliced

- 2oz lean turkey breast

- 2 turkey bacon, cooked

- 2 green lettuce leaves

Note: This recipe is good for one, adjust accordingly.

Procedure:

1. Simply layer the meats, tomato slices, and lettuce between the toast and you're good to go.

Healthy Mini Egg Omelet
Ingredients:

- 4 cups broccoli

- 4 whole eggs

- 1 cup egg whites

- ¼ cup low-fat cheddar cheese, shredded

- ¼ cup pecorino Romano cheese, shredded

- Salt and pepper to taste

- Cooking spray

Note: This recipe makes 4 mini omelets. Double the portions if you need more.

Procedure:

1. Preheat oven to 350°.

2. Steam the broccoli in water for 6 to 7 minutes. When cooked, crush into smaller pieces.

3. Add olive oil and season with salt and pepper.

4. Spray a standard non-stick cupcake molder with cooking spray and put broccoli mixture evenly into 9 molds.

5. In a mixing bowl, beat whole eggs, egg whites and grated pecorino Romano cheese. Add salt and pepper to taste. Pour over the broccoli mixture until mold is ¾ full.

6. Top each with grated cheddar cheese.

7. Bake for at least 20 minutes.

8. Serve immediately. If you have leftovers, wrap them in plastic wrap or put in a zip-lock plastic bag and refrigerate. It is good for one week.

Special Breakfast Enchilada

Ingredients:

- 3 cups egg whites (from about 18 large eggs)

- 2 tbsp water

- Salt and pepper to taste

- Cooking spray

- 1 tsp olive oil

- ½ cup chopped scallions

- 1 medium diced tomatoes

- 2 tbsp chopped cilantro

- 10 oz pack frozen spinach

- 4.5 oz can chopped green chilis

- Salt and pepper to taste

- ½ cup grated cheese

- 1 cup green enchilada sauce

- 1 medium avocado, diced

Note: This recipe yields 6 servings.

Procedure:

1. Preheat oven to350°F.

2. Pour in 1/ cup enchilada sauce on the bottom of a baking dish (9x12 inches).

3. In a mixing bowl, beat egg whites, add water, and a pinch of salt and pepper.

4. Coat a non-stick pan with cooking spray and set stove to medium heat.

5. Add ½ cup of the egg whites, swirl evenly to cover the entire pan. Cook for about 2 minutes and then flip to cook the other side. Set aside and repeat with the remaining egg whites. You should be able to make 6 "egg tortillas".

6. Heat oil in another non-stick pan and set to medium heat. Cook the scallions for about 2 to 3 minutes. Add tomato and cilantro. Add salt and pepper to taste and cook for another 1 minute. Add in spinach and green chili and let it cook for another 5 minutes. Adjust seasoning according to your preference.

7. Remove from heat and add ½ cup of cheese and mix well.

8. Divide spinach among the "egg tortillas". Roll up and place each side down in the baking dish. Top the "tortillas" with your remaining enchilada sauce and cheese. Cover the baking dish with foil and bake until cheese is melted, which will take about 20 to 25 minutes.

9. You can serve topped with diced scallions and avocados.

Bacon-Wrapped Mini Meatloaf

Ingredients:

- 1 lb lean ground beef

- ½ lb bacon, cut in chunks

- 8 strips of bacon (do not cut)

- ¼ cup coconut milk

- 2 cloves minced garlic

- ½ cup minced fresh chives

- Chopped, fresh parsley

- Ground black pepper

Note: This recipe serves 4 people.

Procedure:

1. Preheat oven to 400°F.

2. In a mixing bowl, mix ground beef, bacon chunks, garlic, chives, and coconut milk. Season with ground black pepper. Bacon replaces salt.

3. Put one bacon slice each on a medium-sized muffin molder, creating rings.

4. Fill the rings with the mixed beef.

5. Cook in the oven for about 30 minutes.

6. Remove the mini meatloaf and top with parsley.

7. This is a good low-carb day breakfast.

Low-Carb Egg Benedict Breakfast

Ingredients:

- 2 tbsp butter

- 1 beaten egg

- 1 slice ham

- Lazy hollandaise sauce

For Hollandaise Sauce

- ¼ cup mayonnaise

- 1 tsp lemon or lime juice

- ¼ tsp pepper

Note: This recipe is good for one; adjust if serving 2 or more.

Procedure:

1. In a small non-stick skillet, heat butter and add egg. Allow the egg to form into a solid mass; if you have an "egg ring", it is perfect for this. Flip to cook the other side.

2. Let the egg cool for about 2 to 3 minutes.

3. With the use of a regular drinking glass or a circle cookie cutter, cut the ham to fit the scrambled eggs' diameter. You might need to fold the cooked egg several times to create a layer.

4. Cut the cooked egg to look like a muffin and place on top of the ham.

5. Top with hollandaise sauce.

How to Make Hollandaise Sauce

1. Blend all the ingredients for the sauce. Heat before topping onto your egg Benedict.

Avocado Grilled Chicken with Mango Salad

Ingredients:

- 1 lb chicken breast

- 1 cup avocado, diced

- 1 cup mango, diced (1 ½ mangoes)

- 2 tbsp red onion, diced

- 6 cups baby red lettuce

For the Vinaigrette

- 2 tbsp olive oil

- 2 tbsp balsamic vinegar

- Salt and pepper

Procedure:

1. Grill chicken breasts and slice lengthwise. Put in a salad bowl.

2. Whisk together the ingredients for the vinaigrette and set aside.

3. Toss avocado, mango, red onion and sliced chicken breasts.

4. Line a salad platter with the baby lettuce and place the avocado and chicken mixture.

5. Drizzle with the vinaigrette just before serving.

This low-carb chicken salad is not just perfect for breakfast but also for lunch and dinner.

Lunch and Dinner Recipes

3-Flavor Chicken
Ingredients:

- 2 chicken breasts
- Olive oil in a spray bottle
- Baby spinach leaves, blanched
- 1 medium tomato, sliced
- 2 tsp each of tomato, basil, and garlic seasoning

Note: This recipe makes 2 portions; you can double the ingredients to make 4, and so on.

Procedure:

1. Season chicken breasts on both sides.

2. Set a non-stick pan to medium heat and spray olive oil.

3. Add the seasoned chicken breasts and cook on each side.

4. Serve with tomatoes and spinach. You may also sprinkle some oil or seasoning on the veggies.

5. Another option is to season with balsamic vinegar.

Chicken Caribbean

Ingredients:

- 2 chicken breasts (skinless)

- Olive oil in a spray bottle

- 1 tsp low sodium soy sauce

- 1 tsp cider vinegar

- 1 tbsp Caribbean jerk seasoning

- 1 tsp water

Note: This makes 2 servings, adjust accordingly if you want to make more.

Procedure:

- In a zip-lock bag or a container with cover, place all the ingredients. Massage the chicken gently until it is fully coated with marinade.

- Let the marinated chicken sit for at least 30 to 45 minutes.

- Grill the chicken over medium oil. You can also broil if you want to.

- Serve hot with your veggie salad for low-carb days or brown rice for high-carb days.

For more flavorful chicken, you can marinate overnight. You may also keep it in the refrigerator (if you are making a batch) and cook when needed.

Italian Chicken with Herbs

Ingredients:

- 2 chicken breasts, boneless and skinless
- Olive in spray bottle
- A dash of dried red pepper, ground
- 1/3 tsp salt
- ½ tsp Italian seasoning
- 4 tsp red wine vinegar
- 1 tsp water

Note: This recipe makes 2 portions, double the measurements if you are preparing more.

Procedure:

1. In a zip-lock bag (you can also use a container with cover), place all the ingredients. Make sure the chicken is coated with the marinade. Leave for at least 30 minutes. To make it more flavorful, prepare the day before you intend to cook it and just keep in the refrigerator.

2. Grill chicken over medium to high heat, cooking on each side.

3. For a low-carb day, add in your favorite vegetable salad. You can also drizzle the chicken with a few drops of salad dressing.

4. For high-carb days, serve with brown rice and a side dish of steamed veggies.

Lime Chicken with Spices

Ingredients:

- 2 chicken breast halves, boneless and skinless

- 2 tsp butter

- 2 tsp olive oil

- 2 tbsp low sodium chicken broth

- 1 ½ tbsp lime juice

- ¼ tsp salt

- ¼ tsp pepper

- ½ tsp garlic powder

- ¼ tsp onion powder

- A pinch of cayenne pepper

- ، A pinch of paprika

- ¼ tsp thyme

Note: This is good for 2; adjust portioning when you intend to serve more.

Procedure:

1. Mix together the seasonings and the chicken breast in a large zip-lock bag. Make sure that the chicken is well-coated. Let it stand for at least 1 hour to let the flavor set in. If you want to make it more flavorful, marinate the chicken overnight.

2. Set a non-stick skillet to medium heat and put the butter and olive oil.

3. When butter is melted, add in the chicken breasts and cook on each side.

4. Remove from pan and set aside.

5. To the same skillet, add the lime juice and the chicken broth. With the use of a whisk, mix the liquids and continue boiling until sauce is slight reduced.

6. Add the cooked chicken into the skillet and coat with the sauce.

7. Serve with blanched asparagus or broccoli on low-carb days. On the other hand, serve with sweet potatoes on your high-carb days.

8. You may add grated cheese on reward days.

Baked Potatoes and Chicken

This is a complete meal that the whole family will love, whether or not they are also on a diet.

Ingredients:

- 2 chicken breasts, skinless, diced

- 1 lb red potatoes

- Oil in spray bottle

- A bunch of asparagus, trimmed and cut into 1-inch pieces (you can also use red and green bell pepper or any other vegetable you like)

- 1/3 fresh basil, chopped

- 4 gloves of garlic, thinly sliced

- 1 ½ tbsp olive oil

- 1 tsp fresh rosemary, chopped

- A pinch of ground pepper to taste

- ½ cup chicken broth (optional)

Note: This is good for one person only but if you have to prepare for more people, you can adjust measurement accordingly.

Procedure:

1. Preheat oven to 400°.

2. Spray your baking dish with oil and place the chicken breasts, potatoes, tomatoes, vegetables, basil, garlic, olive oil and chicken broth. Sprinkle fresh rosemary and ground pepper.

3. Bake for about 45 minutes, checking and turning occasionally to make sure both sides are cooked.

4. Serve.

High-Carb Chicken and Turkey Medley

Ingredients:

- 2 chicken breasts, boneless and skinless

- 2 slices Turkey bacon slices, diced

- Olive oil in spray bottle

- 1 ½ tsp butter

- ¼ cup apple, diced

- 2 ½ tbsp apple cider

- 1 cup brown rice

- 2 ½ tbsp low-sodium chicken broth

- 1 tsp thyme, dried

- salt and pepper

Note: This recipe serves only 1 person, adjust measurements if preparing for more than 1.

Procedure:

1. Spray oil on a non-stick pan and set to medium heat.

2. Put the chicken breasts to the pan and season with salt and pepper. Cook both sides.

3. Remove cooked chicken from pan and set aside.

4. In the same pan, cook the turkey bacon for about 5 minutes or until it turns brown.

5. Add apple and thyme. Add another pinch of salt and pepper.

6. When the apples turn to brown, bring in the apple cider and chicken broth.

7. Increase to high heat.

8. Let the sauce cook until it thickens, don't forget to stir continuously.

9. Add in butter and let it melt.

10. Next, put back in the pan and coat with the sauce. Simmer for about 2 to 3 minutes.

11. You can serve with brown rice.

12. If you making several batches, you can store in the freezer and simply reheat when needed.

Pork Roast

Ingredients:

- 1 lb pork tenderloin

- 5 gloves of garlic, minced

- 1 tsp dried parsley flakes

- ½ tsp dried thyme leaves

- 1 tsp pepper

- 1 tbsp lemon juice (you can also use lime juice, depending on what's available)

- 1 tsp olive oil

Note: This recipe can serve at least 4 people.

Procedure:

1. Preheat oven at 450°F.

2. Line a roasting pan with foil and spray with oil.

3. In a mixing bowl, combine garlic, parsley, thyme and pepper.

4. In a small cup, put the lemon juice.

5. Brush pork with lemon juice and then rub with the garlic and spice mixture over the top and both its sides. Place in the roasting pan with the garlic and spice marinade side up.

6. Bake for about 35 minutes or until pork is evenly cooked.

7. Let the pork stand for 5 to 10 minutes before cutting and serving.

8. Serve with your favorite vegetable salad.

Healthy Baked Meatballs

Ingredients:

- 16oz ground Turkey meat (93% lean)
- 2 egg whites
- 1/2 cup oatmeal
- ¼ cup nonfat milk
- ½ cup parsley
- 1 tbsp onions, dehydrated flakes
- ½ tsp oregano, ground
- ½ tsp garlic powder

Note: This recipe serves 4 with about 8 meatballs each.

Procedure:

1. Preheat oven at 400°F.

2. Spray a baking dish with oil.

3. In a mixing bowl, combine egg whites, oats and milk. Add in parsley, oregano, onions, garlic power and mix well. Add in ground turkey and mix well.

4. Make about 32 uniform meatballs (about 1 scoop).

5. Line in the baking dish, with a good distance from one another.

6. Bake in the oven for about 7 to 10 minutes or until the inside is cooked.

7. Serve with brown rice for high-carb days or vegetable salad on low-carb days.

Healthy BBQ

Ingredients:

- 1 ¼ lbs boneless pork tenderloin, lean

- Sea salt

- Ground black pepper

- Garlic powder

- ¼ cup and 2 tbsp barbecue sauce (separate)

- Olive oil spray

Note: This BBQ recipe yields 4 servings.

Procedure:

1. Slice pork tenderloin in half, crosswise, and then slice each half lengthwise into quarters, yielding 8 strips. Season slices with sea salt, ground pepper and garlic powder. Place pork in a zip-lock plastic bag. Spoon ¼ cup of BBQ sauce and mix with the pork. Refrigerate overnight.

2. Pre-heat broiler. Line a baking sheet with aluminum foil and lightly spray with oil.

3. Place strips on the baking sheet in a single layer.

4. Broil for 2 to 3 minutes. Flip on the other side and continue to broil for 2 to 3 minutes more.

5. Serve with the sauce dripping. Serve with brown rice for high-carb days and vegetable salad with light dressing on low-carb days.

Delicious Turkey Burger

Ingredients:

- 8 oz raw ground turkey

- Olive oil in a spray bottle

- 1 tsp minced garlic

- ¼ tsp cayenne pepper

- ½ tsp hot sauce (optional)

Note: This recipe serves two persons; you can adjust measurements as needed.

Procedure:

1. In a mixing bowl, combine the ground turkey with cayenne pepper and garlic. Add in the hot sauce if you want. Make sure the turkey and the seasonings are mixed thoroughly. Form into patties.

2. Spray oil in a non-stick pan and set to medium heat. Cook turkey patties on each side.

3. Serve immediately with carrot and celery sticks for low-carb days and boiled red potatoes on high-carb days.

Healthy Steak Tenderloin

Ingredients:

- 6 oz sirloin steak, lean and boneless
- Olive oil in spray bottle
- ¾ steak seasoning
- 1 tsp parsley flakes
- 1 tsp rosemary flakes

Note: This recipe makes 2 servings, you may add portions if you need more.

Procedures:

1. Spray olive oil on each steak.

2. Sprinkle the steaks with seasoning, parsley and rosemary.

3. Grill steak over high heat. You can also cook in a broiler.

4. Serve hot with your favorite greens with light salad dressing on low-carb days. For high-carb days, you can add baked sweet potato or brown rice; and you can still have the veggies as side dish.

Roasted Beef with Stir-Fry Veggies

Ingredients:

- 6 oz lean sirloin steak, boneless
- Olive oil in spray bottle
- 2 tsp low-sodium soy sauce
- ½ tsp cornstarch
- 1/8 ground ginger
- 1 tsp roasted garlic and bell pepper seasoning

- 1/3 cup assorted veggies (you can use snow peas, broccoli, and bell pepper strips)
- 1/3 cup water

Note: This recipe yields 2 portions, double the measurements if you need to make 4.

Procedure:

1. Cut the sirloin steak into 1/4 –inch strips.

2. In a mixing bowl, put the soy sauce, ginger, roasted garlic and bell pepper seasoning, cornstarch and water. Mix thoroughly and set aside.

3. Heat oil on medium to high setting in a non-stick pan. Add beef slices in small batches and cook each for about 5 minutes.

4. Spray more oil if needed.

5. When all the meat slices are done, cook the veggies in the same pan.

6. Serve with almonds or sliced avocado on your low-carb days or with brown rice on high-carb days.

Low-Carb Blue Cheese Steak

Ingredients:

- 6 oz cube steak
- 1/3 cup blue cheese crumbles
- Olive oil in spray bottle
- Red onion, chopped
- ½ tbsp Salt and pepper

Note: This recipe serves 2, double or triple the portions if you need more.

Procedure:

1. Preheat broiler.

2. Heat a non-stick pan over medium heat and spray oil. Add the seasoned meat and cook on each side.

3. Line the broiler pan with foil and place the steak. Top meat with blue cheese and onion.

4. Broil until cheese melts.

5. Serve with steamed greens.

6. If you are making more portions and you want to freeze until you need them, after pan searing the meat, store in a zip-lock plastic and put in the freezer. In a separate zip-lock bag, put onion and blue cheese and freeze as well. You can broil anytime meat is thawed or you can cook it in a microwave oven; just make sure to top the meat with blue cheese and onion.

Sirloin Steak with Veggies

Ingredients:

- 6 oz lean sirloin steak, boneless

- Olive oil in spray bottle

- 1 cup green beans

- 1 medium tomato, chopped

- ¾ tsp garlic, minced

- Salt and pepper to taste

Note: This recipe can serve 1 to 2 persons, if you need to make more portions, adjust the measurements accordingly.

Procedure:

1. In a non-stick pan spray some oil and set stove to high heat. Add meat and cook on each side. Remove from pan and set aside.

2. Adjust heat to medium and in the same pan, add green beans and sauté for 3 minutes and then add garlic and cook for another one minute. Season with salt and pepper.

3. Add diced tomatoes and cook for a minute.

4. Cover pan and let the tomatoes become saucy, about 3 to 4 minutes.

5. Serve the meat with the vegetables on the side.

6. For low-carb days, add sliced avocado; and for high-carb days, serve with baked potato/ sweet potato or brown rice.

Sweet Pork Tenderloin

Ingredients:

- 6 oz lean pork tenderloin
- 1 tbsp honey
- ½ tbsp vinegar
- ¼ tsp vanilla
- 1/8 tsp paprika
- A dash of ground mustard
- Salt and pepper to taste

Note: This makes 2 servings, adjust accordingly if you need more.

Procedure:

1. Combine honey and other flavorings in a zip-lock bag and mix well.

2. Add the pork tenderloin in the zip-lock bag and coat with the honey glaze all over.

3. Heat a non-stick pan over meat settings and cook pork tenderloin on each side.

4. Serve hot with a portion of pecans and vegetable salad on a low-carb day. On the other hand, you can serve it with baked sweet potato or brown rice and side salad for a high-carb day.

Special Tenderloin with Herbs and Spices

Ingredients:

- 6 oz pork tenderloin, lean

- Olive oil in spray bottle

- ½ tsp paprika

- ¼ tsp dried thyme

- ¼ tsp salt

- 1/8 tsp black pepper

Note: The recipe is good for 2 persons so you can adjust measurements when needed.

Procedure:

1. In a mixing bowl, mix all the flavorings and spices. When thoroughly mixed, sprinkle over the pork tenderloins.

2. Spray oil on a non-stick pan and set to medium heat. Add the pork and cook on each side.

3. Serve with your choice of greens for a low-carb day or sweet potato for a high-carb day.

Herbed Roast Pork with Garlic

Ingredients:

- 6 oz lean pork tenderloins

- Olive oil in spray bottle

- 2 tsp roasted garlic and herb seasoning

Note: This is good for 1 to 2 persons so if you need to feed more, adjust measurements.

Procedure:

1. Season pork with the roasted garlic and herb.

2. Spray oil on a non-stick pan and set to medium heat. Cook the pork tenderloin on each side.

3. This is perfect for a low-carb day when you serve with side salad with olive oil and balsamic dressing. If on a high-carb day, you can serve with steamed asparagus and brown rice.

Grilled Chicken Wings

Ingredients:

- 4 pieces chicken wings

- Chicken spice mix seasoning

- Broccoli, asparagus, lettuce (or your choice of greens)

- Salsa

Note: This is good for 1 to 2 persons.

Procedure:

1. Preheat oven to 350°F.

2. Generously coat chicken wings with seasoning, making sure they are completely coated.

Insert chicken wings in the oven and cook until they are golden brown and crunchy.

3. Toss your choice of vegetables and top with salsa.

4. This is good for a low-carb day.

Low-Carb Meatballs Barbecue

Ingredients:

- 1 lb ground pork, lean
- 1 tsp granulated sugar substitute
- 1 tsp paprika
- ½ tsp salt
- ¼ tsp black pepper
- ¼ tsp cayenne pepper
- ½ tsp ground cumin
- ¼ tsp celery salt
- 1 medium-sized egg
- ¼ cup almond flour
- 1 tbsp water

For the BBQ Sauce

- ¼ cup yellow mustard
- 2 tsp hot sauce
- 1 tbsp dried onion flakes
- 3 tbsp granulated sugar substitute
- 2 tbsp apple cider vinegar
- 2 tbsp ketchup
- Salt and pepper to taste

Note: This recipe makes 16 meatballs, 4 meatballs per serving.

Procedure:

1. First, mix all the barbecue sauce ingredients in a saucepan, stir until fully mixed and smooth. Over low heat, simmer sauce for about 8 minutes. Set aside.

2. In a mixing bowl, combine all the ingredients for the meatballs and mix. Form into medium-sized balls, this will give you 16 pieces.

3. In a non-stick skillet, fry meatballs over medium heat. Cooking time is 3 to 4 minutes on each side.

4. Toss the cooked meatballs into the barbecue sauce. Once meatballs are fully coated, spread them on a baking dish lined with parchment paper. Broil for about 2 to 3 minutes.

5. Serve with coleslaw or your favorite greens.

Low-Carb Roasted Turkey

Ingredients:

- 1 whole turkey
- 1 tbsp vegetable oil
- 1 tsp Italian seasoning
- Salt and pepper

Note: This yields at least 18 servings.

Procedure:

1. Preheat your outdoor grill to get medium to high heat.

2. Prepare the turkey. After washing it clean, pat to dry. Turn the wings back so the neck skin is held in place. Turn the legs to a tucked position.

3. Brush turkey skin with oil. Season both inside and out with the Italian seasoning, salt and pepper.

4. Position the turkey, with the breast side up, on the metal grate inside a large roasting pan. Place the pan on the prepared grill.

5. Cooking time is 2 to 3 hours.

6. Remove from the grill and let it stand for about 15 minutes before carving the turkey.

7. Serve with your favorite greens.

Delicious Salmon Fillet with Herbs and Spices

Ingredients:

- 4 pieces salmon fillet, no bones and skin
- ½ cup melted unsalted butter
- 2 tbsp ground paprika
- 1 tbsp ground cayenne pepper
- 1 tbsp onion powder
- 2 tsp salt
- ½ tsp ground white pepper
- ½ tsp ground black pepper
- ¼ tsp dried thyme
- ¼ tsp dried basil
- ¼ tsp dried oregano

Note: This recipe yields 4 servings.

Procedure:

1. In a mixing bowl, mix the spices: paprika, cayenne pepper, salt, onion powder, white and black pepper, basil, thyme and oregano.

2. Brush each salmon fillet with ¼ of the butter and evenly sprinkle with the mixed spices.

3. Drizzle on each side with half of the remaining butter.

4. Heat a large skillet to high and cook salmon, with the butter side down, until crust is blackened; this will take about 2 to 5 minutes.

5. Turn the fillet and drizzle with the last remaining butter.

6. Continue cooking until crust is blackened. It is ready when fish is flaked when you poke with a fork.

Spicy Pork Tenderloin

Ingredients:

- 6 oz pork tenderloin
- 1 tsp butter
- Olive oil in spray bottle
- ½ tsp paprika
- ¼ dried oregano
- ½ tsp garlic powder
- ½ tsp ground cumin
- ¾ tsp salt
- 1/8 tsp fennel seeds
- A dash of ground cayenne pepper
- ¼ cup chicken broth

Note: This recipe makes 2 servings.

Procedure:

1. In a small mixing bowl, combine all the herbs and spices.

2. Brush half of the spice on one side of the tenderloin.

3. Set non-stick pan to medium heat and add the pork, with the spiced side down. While pork is cooking in that position, sprinkle the rest of the spices on top.

4. Cook on each side until browned.

5. Remove from pan and keep the pork warm.

6. On the same pan, add butter and whisk all the browned bits and spices left in the pan. Turn the heat to medium-high and add the chicken broth. Continue whisking until sauce is reduced by half.

7. Place the pork on a serving plate and drizzle the sauce on top.

8. Serve with your potato salad or baked potato for a high-carb day or your favorite greens for a low-carb day.

Easy Garlic and Herb Shrimp Salad

Ingredients:

- 25 pieces large shrimps, peeled and deveined
- Olive oil in a spray bottle
- 2 tsp roasted garlic and herb seasoning
- Raw baby spinach

Note: This makes 2 servings.

Procedure:

1. Thoroughly season shrimp with roasted garlic and herb mix.

2. Spray oil on a non-stick pan and set to medium heat.

3. Cook shrimp.

4. Serve immediately over a bed of baby spinach. You can toss spinach with balsamic vinegar and olive oil before adding the shrimp.

Perfect Salmon Fillet

Ingredients:

- 8 oz salmon fillet
- ½ tbsp butter
- 1 tbsp Cajun seasoning
- 1 tsp minced garlic

- 2 tbsp balsamic vinegar

- 2 lemon wedges

Note: Makes 2 servings. Add portions to make more.

Procedure:

1. Heat a non-stick pan set at medium heat. Melt butter and add salmon. Cook on each side but you have to be careful because salmon cooks rather quickly. If salmon is overcooked, it becomes dry.

2. Remove fish from pan and keep warm.

3. On the same pan, add in the rest of the butter, then add garlic and Cajun seasoning.

4. Cook for about 2 minutes before adding the balsamic vinegar. Simmer for another 2 minutes, with continuous stirring.

5. Put back the salmon to the pan and finish the cooking process.

6. Place the fillet on a serving plate and garnish with lemon wedges.

7. Serve with steamed asparagus or baby spinach if you are on a low-carb day. When you are on a high-carb day, add brown rice.

Chapter 8 Meal plan

Another important aspect of the carb cycling diet plan is to know how to tweak the plan to suit your individual needs and personal objectives.

First, you need to know how to calculate your daily carb needs.

How to Calculate Your Daily Carb Needs

Under the carb cycling diet plan, the days are broken into two categories:

The High carb days

The Low carb days

Therefore, to calculate your carb needs for both low and high carb days, you should use this formula:

Men

High carb day

2–3 grams of carbs (x your body weight in pounds)

1–1.25 grams of protein (x your body weight in pounds)

0-0.15 grams of fat (x your body weight in pounds)

Low carb day

0.5–1.5 grams of carbs (x your bodyweight in pounds)

1.25–1.5 grams of protein (x your bodyweight in pounds)

0.15–0.35 grams of fat (x your bodyweight in pounds)

Women

High carb day

About 1 gram of carbs (x your bodyweight in pounds)

0.75 grams of protein (x your bodyweight in pounds)

0-0.15 grams of fat (x your body weight in pounds)

Low carb day

0.2–0.5 grams of carbs (x your bodyweight in pounds)

About 1 gram of protein (x your bodyweight in pounds)

0.1–0.2 grams of fat (x your bodyweight in pounds)

So a man who weighs 150 pounds would have the following meal allowances on high carb days;

Men

High Carb Days

2–3 grams of carbs (x 150) =300-450g

1–1.25 grams of protein (x 150) = 150-187.5g

0-0.15 grams of fat (x 150) =0-22.5g

Low Carb Days

0.5–1.5 grams of carbs (x 150) = 75 - 225g

1.25–1.5 grams of protein (x 150) = 187.5 – 225g

0.15–0.35 grams of fat (x 150) = 22.5 – 52.5g

A Woman who weighs 200 pounds would have the following allowances:

Woman

Low Carb Days

0.2–0.5 grams of carbs (x 200) = 40-100g

About 1 gram of protein (x 200) = 200g

0.1–0.2 grams of fat (x 200) = 20 -40g

Woman

High Carb Days

About 1 gram of carbs (x 200) = 200g

0.75 grams of protein (x 200) = 150g

0-0.15 grams of fat (x 200) = 0-30g

How to Calculate Your Daily Caloric Requirement

The next thing you should know is how to calculate your daily caloric requirements.

Each person has their own unique estimated daily calorie maintenance level, which is the amount of calories your body requires daily. However, to lose weight, you need to create a calorie deficit in order to force your body to go into its energy store to get the extra calories it needs.

There are many calculators online that you can use to easily determine your daily calorie requirement but you can also calculate it manually using this simple formula.

Current body weight in pounds X 14

Current body weight in Pounds X 17

Your estimated daily calorie requirement would fall somewhere between these two amounts.

So let's say you currently weigh 150 pounds, your daily calorie maintenance level would fall between 1,200 and 2,550.

150 X 14 = 1,200

150 X 17 = 2,550

If you use this formula, you should try to stick with the lower values because many other factors like your age, sex, activity levels, metabolic rates, and height also have roles to play in determining daily calorie maintenance level.

Sample Meal Plan

Here is a sample meal plan to give you an idea of what your meal plan should look like on the carb cycling diet.

	High Carb Day	**Low Carb Day**
Breakfast	Egg Whites, Cereal, skim milk, blueberries.	Whole eggs, egg whites, oatmeal, skim milk
Mid-Morning Snack	Whey protein, medium-sized banana.	Whey protein, Peanut butter, Skim milk
Lunch	Chicken breast, brown rice, free-fat mayonnaise.	Deli turkey slices, whole wheat bread, mustard, tomato, lettuce.

Mid-Afternoon Snack	White Tuna, Whole-wheat bread, free- fat mayonnaise.	Greek Yoghurt, Sliced almonds.
Snack	Whole wheat bagel, fat-free cream cheese, Gatorade.	
Dinner	Lean Sirloin steak, Broccoli, mixed green salad with fat-free salad dressing, sweet potato	Tilapia, Brown rice, green salad, brown rice.
Late Night Snack	Casein protein	Peanut butter, whey protein.

Conclusion

Thank you again for downloading this book!

I hope I was able to teach you to learn and understand the intricacies of the carbs cycling diet, recipes and other related concepts under this specific diet program.

By doing this, you will start to enjoy the benefits of having a healthy lifestyle through a balanced diet and regulated exercise routines. This may not be an easy weight management journey at first. However, through constant practice and proper motivation, you will eventually have that body physique and that optimal state of health that you have desired for the longest time. You just have to keep going even if the diet program seems tough.

Thank you and good luck!

CPSIA information can be obtained
at www.ICGtesting.com
Printed in the USA
LVHW01s1533181117
556808LV00028B/630/P